Movement Related Cortical Potentials Based Brain Computer Interface for Stroke Rehabilitation

Movement Related Cortical Potentials Based Brain Computer Interface for Stroke Rehabilitation

PhD Thesis by

Imran Khan Niazi

Center for Sensory-Motor Interaction (SMI),
Department of Health Science and Technology,
Aalborg University, Aalborg, Denmark

River Publishers

Aalborg

ISBN 978-87-92982-45-2 (paperback)
ISBN 978-87-92982-33-9 (e-book)

Published, sold and distributed by:
River Publishers
P.O. Box 1657
Algade 42
9000 Aalborg
Denmark

Tel.: +45369953197
www.riverpublishers.com

Table of contents

Acknowledgments

The Ph.D. thesis describes the work carried out at the Center for Sensory-Motor Interaction (SMI), Aalborg University, Denmark in the period from 2009 to 2012.

This thesis would not have been possible without the support and encouragement of some people that I would like to mention here.

I especially want to thank my supervisor *Professor Dario Farina*, whose encouragement, supervision and support from an idea to the final stage enabled me to develop an understanding of this topic. I appreciated that he was always accessible and willing to discuss and explore new ideas.

I further want to express my gratitude to Head of the Department *Associate Professor Kim Dremstrup*, who gave me the opportunity to carry out this research at Aalborg University by hiring me as a PhD student to start with and later on for his continuous moral and financial support, which was essential in completion of this thesis.

My sincere thanks to *Associate Professor Natalie Mrachacz-Kersting* helping me understand neurophysiological aspects of the project and specially for assisting me in the lab.

My special thanks to *Ning Jiang* and *Thomas Lorrain* for helping me in enhancing my capabilities with Matlab. Without their support, it would have been a difficult journey. It was always a pleasure to discuss the technical aspect of the projects with both of them, which often resulted in making life easier.

I would also like to thank all my colleagues at SMI for creating an inspiring and positive working environment. In particular, I would like to thank *Signe Rom Kristensen*. She was always available to discuss ideas, especially in listening my frustration and helping me to get out of those difficult phases. I would like to thanks also *Mads Jochumsen* for his support during the last two years.

Last but not least, I would like to thank my family, my parents *Umer Hayat Khan Niazi* and *Gohar Anjum Niazi*, brother *Muhammad Nauman Khan Niazi* for their encouragement and believe in me and especially my wife *Kalsoom Bibi* for her never ending support in good and bad days. During my PhD, we were blessed with the most precious gift of our lives,

viii   MRCP based brain computer interface for stroke rehabilitation

our son *Muhammad Taha Khan Niazi*. Thanks to his innocent smiles which makes me forget the tiredness of the office in the later days of my PhD.

Thanks to Almighty God above all!

Imran Khan Niazi
Aalborg, Denmark , 2012

List of articles

The Ph.D. thesis is based on four articles:

I. Imran Khan Niazi, Aleksandra Pavlovic, Sasa Radovanovic, Ning Jiang, Viladmir Kostic, Kim Dremstrup, Dario Farina, Natalie Mrachacz-Kersting. **Inducing plasticity in chronic stroke patients with precise temporal association between cortical potentials and sensory afferent feedback**(In preparation).

II. Imran Khan Niazi, Ning Jiang, Olivier Tiberghien, Jørgen Feldbæk Nielsen, Kim Dremstrup, and Dario Farina. **Detection of movement intention from single-trial movement-related cortical potentials.** *Journal of Neural Engineering*, vol. 8, pp. 066009, 2011.

III. Imran Khan Niazi, Natalie Mrachacz-Kersting, Ning Jiang, Kim Dremstrup, and Dario Farina. **Peripheral electrical stimulation triggered by self-pace detection of motor intention enhances motor evoked potentials.**
IEEE Transactions on Neural Systems and Rehabilitation Engineering, 2012 Jul; 20(4):595-604. (Epub ahead of print), Apr 25. 2012.

IV. Imran Khan Niazi, Ning Jiang, Mads Jochumsen, Jørgen Feldbæk Nielsen, Kim Dremstrup, and Dario Farina. **Detection of movement-related cortical potentials based on subject-independent training.** *Journal of Medical & Biological Engineering & Computing.* (Epub ahead of print) Dec 2012.

Abstract

A brain-computer interface (BCI) is a system that interprets brain signals generated by the user, allowing specific commands from the brain to be sent to an external device. Such interface enables severely disabled people to interact with their environment without the need for any activation of their normal pathways involved in motor commands. The combination of rehabilitation paradigms and BCIs, both of which exploit cortical plasticity, could help people become "able" once again. For this reason, BCI systems appear promising rehabilitation tools.

The aim of this PhD thesis is to study how a BCI system can be used for stroke rehabilitation when it is based on neuromodulation techniques using Hebbian plasticity and movement related cortical potentials (MRCP) with an optimum number of EEG electrodes. Four studies were conducted to achieve this goal: In STUDY I the novel protocol developed in Mrachacz-Kersting et al. 2012 had showed improvement in some relevant clinical measures used to access functionality of motor tasks in stroke population, when applied three times in a week as a training paradigm. These encouraging results from our first study alongside the Mrachacz-Kersting et al. 2012 study served as the basis for development of a self-paced BCI system for induction of plasticity. In STUDY II (pseudo online) detector for self-paced BCI system, based on movement intention detection from initial negative phase of MRCP, was proposed and tested in healthy volunteers and then in STUDY III real online self-paced BCI system for induction of plasticity was implemented and tested. In STUDY IV a subject independent detector (based on STUDY II) was developed and compared with individualized detector. The results were promising as difference between performances of two approaches was not significantly different.

Danish Abstract

Et hjerne-computer interface (BCI) er et system, der fortolker hjernesignaler genereret af specielle kommandoer fra hjernen, som bliver sendt til et eksternt apparat. Dette interface gør alvorligt skadede personer i stand til at interagere med deres omgivelser uden brug af de normale nervebaner, der er involveret i motoriske kommandoer. Kombinationen af rehabiliteringsparadigmer og BCI, der begge inducerer kortikal plasticitet, kan hjælpe personer med at 'blive i stand til' igen. Derfor lader det til, at et BCI-system er et lovende værktøj indenfor rehabilitering.

Målet med denne PhD-afhandling er at undersøge, hvordan et BCI-system kan bruges i rehabilitering af slagtilfælde, når det er baseret på neuromodulationsteknikker, der gør brug af Hebbian plasticitet og bevægelsesrelaterede kortikale potentialer (MRCP), samt et optimalt antal elektroder. Fire studier blev lavet for at opnå dette mål. I STUDIE 1 viste anvendelse af en nye TMS-baseret intervention, beskrevet i Mrachacz-Kersting et al. 2012, forbedringer i relevante kliniske mål af funktionaliteten af motoriske opgaver hos patienter med slagtilfælde, når interventionen blev udført tre gange i løbet af en uge som et træningsparadigme. Disse opmuntrende resultater fra det første studie ledte til udviklingen af et BCI-system, styret i brugerens eget tempo (asynkron), til at inducere plasticitet. I STUDIE 2 blev en (pseudo realtid) detektor for et asynkront BCI-system, baseret på en bevægelsesintention fra den initiale negative fase af MRCP'et, lavet og testet i raske forsøgspersoner, og i STUDIE 3 blev et realtid asynkront BCI-system, til at inducere plasticitet, implementeret og testet. I STUDIE 4 blev en forsøgspersonuafhængig detektor udviklet (baseret på STUDIE 2) og sammenlignet med en individualiseret detektor. Resultaterne er lovende, da forskellen mellem præstationerne af de to fremgangsmåder ikke var signifikant forskellige.

1. Introduction

Stroke is the second leading cause of death and acquired disability in adults worldwide, and therefore it also constitutes a major health care cost (Endres et al. 2011). The world health organization (WHO) estimates that the absolute number of first-ever stroke patients in the European Union and selected European Fair Trade Association Countries will increase from 1.1 million in 2000 to 1.5 million in 2025, if incidence rates remain stable (Truelsen et al. 2006). By 2030, it is estimated that almost 23.6 million people will die from cardio vascular diseases (CVD's), mainly comprising heart disease and stroke (WHO 2012). Following a stroke, many patients unfortunately suffer an additional stroke. Recurrent strokes account for approximately 25% of the total (Burn et al. 1994). The improvement of both primary and secondary stroke rehabilitation and prevention is therefore very important. The consequences after a stroke can be very limiting for both the individual and the family, due to long-term impairments, limited activities (disability) and reduced participation (handicap).

In general, there are two stages of treatment for stroke survivors. These are acute/intensive care and post-stroke rehabilitation. In acute stroke treatment, the stroke itself needs to be terminated to minimize the damage. Intensive care is subsequently required to prevent further damage to the unaffected portions of the brain, and to prevent complications (Gillen et al. 2004). In post-stroke rehabilitation, the aim is to restore or improve body functions so that the stroke survivor becomes as independent as possible, for instance, by motivating the patient to relearn basic skills. The primary means of rehabilitation include physical therapy, occupational therapy, and speech/audiology therapy. Physical therapy helps to restore the physical functioning and skills of the patients, such as walking. The major impairments that physical therapy aims to improve include partial or one-sided paralysis, faulty balance and foot drop. Occupational therapy involves relearning the skills needed for everyday living such as eating, dressing and taking care of oneself. In speech and audiology therapy, stroke survivors are assisted in problems with communication, swallowing or hearing (Gillen et al. 2004).

Currently, there is a plethora of intervention strategies being analyzed, which are also being used to rehabilitate stroke survivors. Examples include pharmacotherapy, physical therapy, functional electrical stimulation and virtual reality therapy (Langhorne et al. 2009). The multitude of strategies available, coupled with the heterogeneity of stroke types, helps to explain why no single intervention has emerged as the most effective. Undoubtedly, as the number of research groups within the field grows and the evidence from scientific experiments amounts, deciding on which rehabilitation path to take for a given stroke patient will improve the rehabilitation outcomes. In recent years, besides classical methods, some artificial methods based on neuromodulation have gained much attention for rehabilitation purposes. An interesting novel idea for delivering artificial stimuli is to trigger such stimuli by decoding the movement intentions of the patients, i.e. by establishing an interface between the patient's brain and external devices for peripheral stimulation. Such interface can be obtained by recording the Electroencephalographic (EEG) signal and is referred to as a brain-computer interface (BCI).

Since Hans Berger's EEG experiments on humans in the early twentieth century (Berger 1929), the idea of reading thoughts from the brain activity has fascinated many scientists. The EEG discovery enabled researchers to measure and start trying to decode the human's brain activity. However, it was only in 1973 that the first prototype of a BCI emerged, developed by Vidal (Vidal 1973). Since the 1990s, BCI research into brain activity as a communication or control channel for external devices has grown exponentially worldwide, resulting in numerous BCI prototypes and applications (Daly et al. 2009, Rebsamen et al. 2007, Birbaumer et al. 2000), but also in the fields of multimedia and virtual reality (Krepki et al. 2007).

1.1 BRAIN-COMPUTER INTERFACES (BCI)

Designing a BCI is a complex task that requires multidisciplinary skills from the engineering and medical fields. A BCI can be formally defined as a "communication and control channel that does not depend on the brain's normal output channels of peripheral nerves and muscles" (Wolpaw et al. 2002). The messages and commands sent through a BCI are encoded into the user's brain activity, meaning that a BCI user 'produces' different mental states (generating

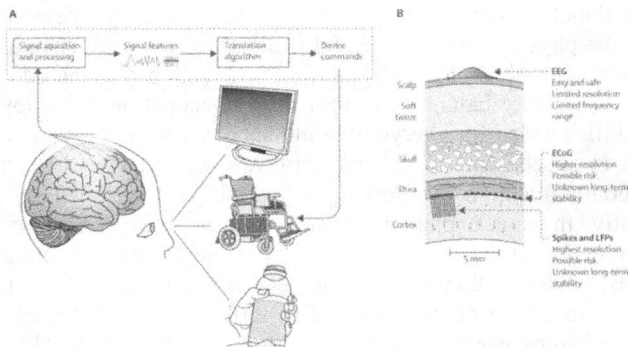

Figure 1: General architecture of a brain-computer interface. (Daly & Wolpaw, 2008).

given neurophysiological signals) while their brain activity is being measured and processed by the system.

The development of a BCI must follow a closed-loop process, generally composed of six parts: brain activity measurement invasively or non-invasively, preprocessing, feature extraction from acquired brain signals, classification/detection of the user intention, and translation into a command to external device and feedback (Figure 1). Traditionally, the different BCI systems are divided into several categories. Among these categories are dependent/independent BCI, invasive/non-invasive BCI, and synchronous/ asynchronous (self-paced) BCI.

1.2 DEPENDENT VERSUS INDEPENDENT BCI

A BCI system does not send the commands to control a computer through the brain's normal output pathways (Cabrera 2009). According to whether or not the subject uses muscle or nerve activity to produce brain activity, the BCI system is considered either dependent or independent. A dependent BCI requires a certain level of motor control from the subject, whereas an independent BCI does not require any motor control. In order to assist and help severely disabled people who do not have any motor control, a BCI must be independent. However, a dependent BCI can be of interest for healthy people, such as for playing video games.

1.3 INVASIVE VERSUS NON-INVASIVE BCI

A BCI system is classified as an invasive or non-invasive BCI according to the way the brain activity is being measured within the BCI (Wolpaw et al. 2002). If the sensors used for measurement are placed within the brain, the BCI is said to be invasive. On the contrary, if the measurement sensors are placed outside the head, on the scalp, the BCI is said to be non-invasive. Invasive recordings either measure the brain's electrical activity on the surface of the cortex (electrocorticography, ECoG) or within the cortex (action potentials or local field potentials, LFP). Non-invasive recordings are obtained as electrical activity from the scalp (electroencephalogram, EEG), magnetic field fluctuation (magneto encephalogram, MEG), metabolic changes (functional magnetic resonance imaging, fMRI, or near infrared spectroscopy, NIRS). Each recording technology has its advantages and limitations with respect to spatial and temporal resolution, portability and cost and risks for the user. As a consequence, a vast majority of current BCI research focuses on EEG signals, as they offer high temporal resolution, are low cost and risk, and are portable (Soekadar 2011).

1.4 SYNCHRONOUS VERSUS ASYNCHRONOUS (SELF-PACED) BCI

Synchronous BCI systems are cue-based, meaning that they depend on a protocol that determines the onset, offset and duration of the operations. For example, a subject might be instructed to move a screen cursor horizontally to the left or right, according to the position of a target. Imaginary movements of the right hand will move the cursor to the right, and imagination of left hand movements moves the cursor to the left. The appearance of the target informs the subject as to the task they are required to perform, a few seconds after the appearance of the cursor the subject is warned to start the task that will produce the desired EEG activity. After a period of time a decision is made by the system on the imagined task (left or right), followed by feedback to the subject about his/her performance. Conversely, an asynchronous (self-paced) BCI is always active. Besides reacting to the pre-determined mental tasks that control the system, it is also able to identify a rest or idle state. In the rest state, the subject does not intend to control the system and therefore the system does not react or give feedback to the subject.

1.5 BRAIN SIGNALS USED IN BCI

BCI aims to identify the brain activity of subjects by having them performing tasks with specific neurophysiological signals (such as brain activity patterns), so that commands can be associated with each of these signals. Several kinds of mental activities may be used to implement a BCI system, and they can be divided into two main groups according to how they are generated. In the first group, subject perceives a specific external stimulus that generates an evoked potential (EP, such as visual evoked potentials). In the second group, there is no external stimulation and the commands are voluntarily generated by the user. This follows an internal cognitive process called spontaneous signals (for instance, slow cortical potentials, sensorimotor rhythms and non-motor cognitive tasks).

In this first category the main signals used in BCIs are the Steady State Evoked Potentials (SSEP) and the P300 (Müller-Putz et al. 2008, Donchin et al. 2000). The main advantage of EP is that, contrary to spontaneous signals, evoked potentials do not require specific user training, as they are automatically generated by the brain in response to a stimulus. Nevertheless, as these signals are evoked, they require external stimulations which can be uncomfortable, cumbersome or tiring for the user. Within the category of spontaneous signals, sensorimotor rhythms (SMR) are widely used, such as event-related de/synchronization (ERD/ERS) (Neuper et al. 2009, Pfurtscheller et al. 1997). Less commonly used neurophysiological signals include slow cortical potentials, such as movement related potentials (MRP), (Do Nascimento 2005) and non-motor cognitive signals, for instance auditory or spatial navigation imagery (Cabrera 2009). In this PhD, the brain signals which have been investigated and discussed are a type of slow cortical potentials, namely the movement-related cortical potentials (MRCPs).

1.5.1   Movement Related Cortical Potentials (MRCP)

The execution of a given motor task is accompanied by a characteristic pattern of EEG potentials - the MRCP. As Do Nascimento (2005) has mentioned, these have been defined as a series of potentials, including the:
1. Readiness Potential (RP), the slow decrease of a brain potential at least 500 ms prior to voluntary movement;
2. Motor Potential (MP), a negative potential following the RP approximately 150 ms prior the onset of a voluntary movement;
3. Movement Monitoring Potential (MMP), a complex negative-positive potential following the onset of a given voluntary motor task.

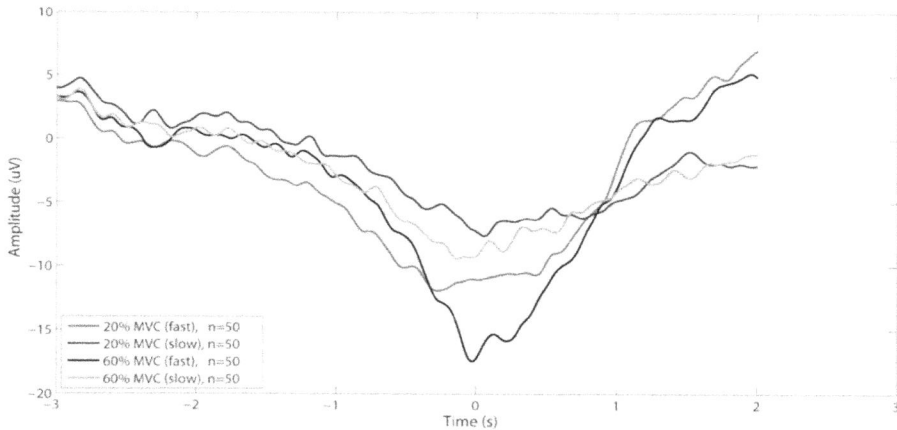

Figure 2: EEG grand average data from large laplacian CZ electrode while performing four different tasks. Time 0 is defined as the movement onset.

MRCPs are present even in the execution of imaginary motor tasks. For example, if the subject imagines a movement, a slow decrease of a brain potential will be visible in the EEG.   Moreover, they reflect the movement's rate of torque development (Figure 2) and its speed (slow, and fast). As the first part of the MRCP occurs before the actual movement, this signal can be used for detection of both imaginary and real movements with short latency.

1.6 BCI AND REHABILITATION

In the rehabilitation approach, a BCI system becomes a neuromodulatory system - a system in which neural functions are modulated by feedback triggered by the decoded brain activity. In order to use a BCI, a new skill must be learned so as to control brain activity to achieve the desired command, and alter the plasticity of the brain. This may take a long period of training for both the subject and the machine learning algorithms (Kennedy et al. 2000). Rehabilitation through BCI control-driven paradigms are based on the capability of learning to modify the efficacy of spared neural ensembles, such as those involved in movement, sensation and cognition, through progressive practice with feedback and reward (Dobkin 2004). In this thesis, neuromodulatory BCI are defined as BCI systems specifically designed and optimized for inducing neuroplasticity. For these systems, the task of designing the feedback and its timing is very important in order to drive specific (rather than unspecific) cortical changes (for example, an increase in the excitability of a specific cortical area).

Thus, learning processes are activated by cognitive and sensory experiences related to feedback from the environment and these are the important factors in inducing cortico-spinal excitability and modifications of brain circuitries. Brain adaptation which occurs due to any damage (stroke etc.) can also be considered as a learning process: thus the brain, although damaged, triggers a reorganization of its structure. Addressing issues concerning brain structure modification, and learning capacity due to brain insults, is very important for an effective translation of neuroscience results into rehabilitation (Kleim et al. 2008).

Jackson et al (Jackson et al. 2001) proposed a model for utilizing the motor imagery in rehabilitation. They proposed that three elements contribute to the rehabilitative outcome: physical execution (musculo-skeletal activity), declarative knowledge (information about the skill the patient has to learn) and non-conscious processes. Definitely, because of the interaction among these three components, the outcome improves with physical execution, but this is not always possible or may be difficult in patients with brain damage. Thus, motor imagery could be helpful for such cases (Jackson et al. 2001). Moreover, the lack of motor execution stresses the role of declarative knowledge and could also be important in disclosing non-conscious aspects of motor learning (Jackson et al. 2001 & 2006).

A closed-loop BCI system uses two types of feedback: sensory and/or visual. These types of feedback can be given in various ways. For example, sensory feedback can be delivered as electrical or tactile stimulation, whereas visual feedback can be given by moving a cursor on a computer screen or through virtual reality. These forms of feedback are provided in real time, showing the subjects how they are performing as a response to specific brain activity. Closed-loop BCI may change cortical excitability because of plasticity in the brain areas. Plasticity is based on the causal association between pre- and post-synaptic connection. According to the Hebbian rule (Hebb 1949), synapses increase their efficacy if the pre-synaptic neuron consistently assists the post-synaptic target neuron to generate action potentials (Sejnowski 1999). One aspect in Hebbian learning relates to the temporal nature of inputs to neuronal synapses, meaning both pre- and post-synaptic neurons have to be active in order to induce a strengthening of the synapse (Gerstner et al. 2002).

1.6.1   Methods to artificially induce plasticity

Plasticity in the human motor cortex can be elicited with various interventions. For example, Transcranial Magnetic Stimulation (TMS) has been used (Butefisch et al. 2004) to enhance use-dependent plasticity when applied while the motor cortex is activated during the performance of a training task. Other non-invasive artificial protocols include repetitive transcranial magnetic stimulation (rTMS) (Ziemann 2004) and pair associated stimulation (PAS) (Stefan et al. 2000).

In PAS protocol, electrical stimulation of peripheral nerve is paired with TMS stimuli applied over the motor cortex (Stefan et al. 2002, Stefan et al. 2000).The idea behind applying these artificial inducing plasticity protocol like PAS protocol is two-fold, they can be used to investigate the mechanisms behind the plasticity of central nervous system and also it can be utilized as a rehabilitation tool for patient population e.g. stroke.   The PAS protocol was designed based on the model of associative long term potentiation (LTP) and long term depression (LTD) (Stefan et al. 2002, Stefan et al. 2000). The plastic changes observed after LTP-induction are rapidly developing, long lasting, fully reversible and pathway specific (Bliss et al. 1973). Similarly, when PAS was applied for 30 minutes same changed were observed by Stefan et al. 2000.

This thesis focuses on the induction of plasticity by triggering peripheral electrical stimulation (PES) with motor commands decoded by a BCI system. A novel technique (modified PAS) was presented based on a conditioning protocol for inducing the changes in the excitability of cortical projections to the tibialis anterior (TA) muscle (Mrachacz-Kersting et al. 2012). The conditioning protocols consisted of a single electrical stimuli of the common peroneal nerve (CPN) delivered at motor threshold (MT) paired with cortical potential (Movement related potentials, MRP's) to arrive during i) the preparation phase (CPN+RP), ii) the movement execution phase (CPN+MP) or iii) the movement monitoring phase (CPN+MMP) of the MRCP. A total of 50 pairings were applied in two sets of 25 trials. The mean peak to peak TA motor evoked potential (MEP) amplitude measured prior to and following each intervention was plotted against TMS intensity. This relation was fit with a and the Boltzman sigmoidal function by the Levenberg-Marquard nonlinear, least-mean-squares fit, as previously described (Devanne et al., 1997).

In this study, it was demonstrated that a physiologically generated signal may be used to drive stimulation at a peripheries leading to associative LTP. Generally in PAS studies, when targeting lower limb muscles it requires greater number of paired stimuli (Mrachacz-Kersting et al. 2007 ; Roy et al. 2007) One possible explanation of this in past studies is that TMS has a low spatial resolution (Ziemann et al. 2008). It not only activates the targeted regions in the brain but also activates other nearby regions within range of the TMS coil. In contrast, the origins of the self-generated brain signals are more focal, possibly making them more suitable for Hebbian-based neuroplasticity.

The results also demonstrate the importance of the timing of PES in relation to the different MRP's components and only the intervention where CPN was stimulated in conjunction with MP phase of MRCP led to significant excitability changes. The results also showed that afferent feedback from the periphery is necessary to induce the observed changes as motor imagery or PES alone did not lead to a significant change in excitability which was observed during the control experiments.

2. Thesis objectives

The results of the study by Mrachacz-Kersting et al. 2012 and earlier work in the BCI lab of Aalborg university lead to the work carried out in this thesis, which have potential implications in BCI systems for rehabilitation used for artificially inducing corticospinal plasticity. The aim of this thesis is to test the modified PAS protocol on stroke patients and develop it further in healthy subjects with a BCI system aimed at inducing plastic changes in the central nervous system based on electrical stimulation triggered by MRCPs detected from EEG signals. Four studies were conducted to achieve this goal:

- **STUDY 1** was conducted on stroke patients to observe the efficacy of the protocol (modified PAS) developed in the study by Mrachacz-Kersting et al. 2012, and its functional implications with respect to rehabilitation.
- **STUDY 2** addressed the problem of detecting the movement intention from single trial EEG. For this purpose, the initial negative phase of the MRCP was used. The detection system proposed is needed for implementing the protocol proposed in the first study in a self-paced paradigm.
- **STUDY 3** examined the complete self-paced BCI system for inducing changes in the excitability of the cortical projections to the target muscle in healthy volunteers online.
- **STUDY 4** developed the detection method proposed in Study II without the need for individualized training.

The final outcome of the four studies is an online (Study III), non-invasive self-paced (Study II) BCI system that does not require any training (Study IV) and that control peripheral electrical stimulation based on the detected movement intention.

STUDY I
In Preparation
Inducing plasticity in chronic stroke patients with precise temporal association between cortical potentials and sensory afferent feedback

Imran Khan Niazi[1], Aleksandra Pavlovic[3], Sasa Radovanovic[3], Ning Jiang[4], Viladmir Kostic[3], Kim Dremstrup[1], Dario Farina[2], Natalie Mrachacz-Kersting[1].

Affiliations:
[1]Center for Sensory-Motor Interaction (SMI)
Department of Health Science and Technology
Aalborg University, Aalborg, Denmark
[2] Department of Neurorehabilitation Engineering
Bernstein Focus Neurotechnology Göttingen
Bernstein Center for Computational Neuroscience
University Medical Center Göttingen
Georg-August University, Göttingen, Germany
[3]Neurology Clinic, Clinical Center of Serbia
Faculty of Medicine, University of Belgrade
Dr. Subotica 6
Belgrade, Serbia
[4]Strategic Technology Management, Otto Bock HealthCare GmbH, Duderstadt, Germany

Corresponding author
Natalie Mrachacz-Kersting
Center for Sensory-Motor Interaction (SMI)
Department of Health Science and Technology
Aalborg University
Fredrik Bajers Vej 7 D3
9220 Aalborg Ø
Denmark

STUDY II
Published In: Journal of Neural Engineering
Detection of movement intention from single-trial movement-related cortical potentials

Imran Khan Niazi[1], Ning Jiang [2], Olivier Tiberghien[3], Jørgen Feldbæk Nielsen[4], Kim Dremstrup[1], and Dario Farina[2][§]

Affiliations:
[1]Center for Sensory-Motor Interaction, Department of Health Science and Technology, Aalborg University Denmark
[2]Department of Neurorehabilitation Engineering, Bernstein Center for Computational Neuroscience, University Medical Center Göttingen, Georg-August University, Göttingen, Germany
[3]Institut de Recherche en Communication et Cybernetique de Nantes (IRCCyN)-Centrale Nantes, 1 rue de la Noë,44321 Nantes, France
[4]Hammel Neurorehabilitation and Research Centre, Research Unit, Voldbyvej 15, 8450 Hammel, Denmark

[§]**Corresponding author**
Dario Farina, PhD
Department of Neurorehabilitation Engineering,
Bernstein Center for Computational Neuroscience,
University Medical Center Göttingen,
Georg-August University
Von-Siebold-Str. 4,37075 Göttingen, Germany
Tel: + 49 (0) 551 / 3920100
Fax: + 49 (0) 551 / 3920110

STUDY III
Published In: IEEE Transactions on Neural Systems and Rehabilitation Engineering

Peripheral electrical stimulation triggered by self-pace detection of motor intention enhances motor evoked potentials

Imran Khan Niazi[1], Natalie Mrachacz-Kersting[1], Ning Jiang [2, 3], Kim Dremstrup[1], and Dario Farina[1, 2§]

Affiliations:

[1]Center for Sensory-Motor Interaction, Department of Health Science and Technology, Aalborg University Denmark
[2]Department of Neurorehabilitation Engineering, Bernstein Center for Computational Neuroscience, University Medical Center Göttingen, Georg-August University, Göttingen, Germany
[3]Strategic Technology Management, Otto Bock HealthCare GmbH, Duderstadt, Germany

§**Corresponding author**
Dario Farina, PhD
Department of Neurorehabilitation Engineering,
Bernstein Center for Computational Neuroscience,
University Medical Center Göttingen,
Georg-August University
Von-Siebold-Str. 4,37075 Göttingen, Germany
Tel: + 49 (0) 551 / 3920100
Fax: + 49 (0) 551 / 3920110

STUDY IV
Published In: Medical & Biological Engineering & Computing
Detection of movement related cortical potentials based on subject-independent training

Imran Khan Niazi[1], Ning Jiang [2, 3], Mads Jochumsen[1], Jørgen Feldbæk Nielsen[4], Kim Dremstrup[1], and Dario Farina[1, 2§]

Affiliations:

[1]Center for Sensory-Motor Interaction, Department of Health Science and Technology, Aalborg University Denmark
[2]Department of Neurorehabilitation Engineering, Bernstein Focus Neurotechnology Göttingen, Bernstein Center for Computational Neuroscience, University Medical Center Göttingen, Georg-August University, Göttingen, Germany
[3]Strategic Technology Management, Otto Bock HealthCare GmbH, Duderstadt, Germany
[4]Hammel Neurorehabilitation and Research Centre, Research Unit, Voldbyvej 15, 8450 Hammel, Denmark

§**Corresponding author**
Dario Farina, PhD
Department of Neurorehabilitation Engineering
Bernstein Focus Neurotechnology Göttingen
Bernstein Center for Computational Neuroscience
University Medical Center Göttingen
Georg-August University
Von-Siebold-Str. 4,37075 Göttingen, Germany
Email: dario.farina@bccn.uni-goettingen.de
Tel: + 49 (0) 551 / 3920100
Fax: + 49 (0) 551 / 3920110

3. Conclusion

The design of assistive / restorative BCI systems aimed at rehabilitation of stroke or other neurological disorders has been an exciting emerging field in the last decade. This thesis focused on the artificial induction of plasticity by triggering PES with motor commands decoded by a non-invasive BCI system. BCI can be used for rehabilitation in two ways: by providing command signals for assistive technological devices, or to recover some abilities by following rehabilitation protocols in clinical settings. Assistive technology, e.g. exoskeletons, has been used for the last few decades and in the last decade BCI has been incorporated for commanding assistive devices. In this thesis we aimed at developing a non-invasive restorative BCI.

In the Mrachacz-Kersting et al. 2012 study, a novel conditioning protocol was proposed and evaluated on healthy subjects based on the fact that repeated activation of somatosensory afferents projecting onto M1 has a pivotal role in motor skill learning in monkeys (Pavlides et al. 1993). So, the basic idea was to couple the naturally generated brain activation, e.g. when a person imagines a simple movement, with the afferent inflow through PES in temporal synchrony. This modified PAS protocol showed the changes in excitability of the neural projections connecting the relevant brain areas to the target muscle. One of the intriguing facts about the proposed protocol is that it requires only 50 pairings to observe the reported changes in MEP amplitude, which are fewer in number than those required in conventional PAS protocols (Mrachacz-Kersting et al. 2007, Roy et al. 2007).

There are very few studies on the application of BCI technology in patients with stroke using a multimodal approach, to better the understanding of the correlation between functional recovery and neurophysiological changes (Soekadar 2011). To improve this fact, Study I was conducted with a multimodal approach in a stroke population with the conditioning paradigm proposed by Mrachacz-Kersting et al. 2012. The results were encouraging and some of the clinically relevant functional measurement showed a significant improvement. The first study alongside the earlier study (Mrachacz-Kersting et al. 2012) served as the basic neurophysiological studies to design and develop a restorative non-invasive BCI system. For developing such a system it was required to detect/predict the movement intention in a self-paced BCI environment with short latency. For this purpose, in Study II the initial negative phase of the MRCPs was exploited and a technique based on optimization of spatial filtering for improving the signal to noise ratio (SNR) of EEG signals was proposed and evaluated in a pseudo online manner. With the proposed method, it was possible to detect/predict the movement intention with latency ranging from -100ms to 100ms of movement onset.

The results of study II paved the path for developing a full online non-invasive BCI system for inducing plasticity (Study III). When the movement intention was detected, a PES was triggered (as shown in Study I for a cue-based paradigm). This intervention also modulated the corticospinal excitability of the projection of the target muscle in healthy subjects. In the last study (Study IV), a practical aspect of the BCI based system has been addressed. For classic BCI systems, training data is needed to calibrate the detector/classifier for each subject and for each session. In Study IV, we addressed this issue and proposed a detector approach for which the training of the detector algorithm (Study II) was done on a database of MRCPs rather than on a training set of MRCPs collected from the subject under study. In this way, the training/calibration phase is not done on a subject basis but is obtained through a dataset of pre-recorded signals from a subject population.

This thesis aimed at the design and implementation of a BCI-based system which can send a command signal based on movement intention detection (prediction). The proposed system was used in restorative rehabilitation paradigms. There is an essential difference between "classic" assistive/restorative devices and BCI-based systems: the former depends on the brain's natural output pathways, while the latter require that the central nervous system controls the cortical neurons instead of the spinal motor neurons. In order to achieve a more natural, and therefore reliable, BCI system, it will be more beneficial to shift the control strategy from process-control to goal-selection.

References

[1]   Berger, H. 1929, "Über das Elektroenkephalogramm des Menschen", Archiv für Psychiatrie und Nervenkrankheiten, vol. 87, pp. 527-570.

[2]   Birbaumer, N., Kubler, A., Ghanayim, N., Hinterberger, T., Perelmouter, J., Kaiser, J., Iversen, I., Kotchoubey, B., Neumann, N. & Flor, H. 2000, "The thought translation device (TTD) for completely paralyzed patients", IEEE Transactions on Rehabilitation Engineering, vol. 8, pp. 190-193.

[3]   Bliss, T.V.P. & Lomo, T. 1973, "Long lasting potentiation of synaptic transmission in the dentate area of the anaesthetized rabbit following stimulation of the perforant path", Journal of Physiology, vol. 232, no. 2, pp. 331-356.

[4]   Burn, J., Dennis, M., Bamford, J., Sandercock, P., Wade, D. & Warlow, C. 1994, "Long-term risk of recurrent stroke after a first-ever stroke: The Oxfordshire community stroke project", Stroke, vol. 25, no. 2, pp. 333-337.

[5]   Butefisch, C.M., Khurana, V., Kopylev, L. & Cohen, L.G. 2004, "Enhancing encoding of a motor memory in the primary motor cortex by cortical stimulation.", J Neurophysiol, vol. 91, no. 5, pp. 2110-2116.

[6]   Cabrera, A.R. 2009, Feature extraction and classification for Brain-Computer Interfaces (PhD thesis), Center for Sensory-Motor Interaction (SMI), Department of Health Science and Technology, Aalborg University.

[7]   Daly, J.J., Wolpaw, J. R. 2008, "Brain-computer interfaces in neurological rehabilitation." The Lancet Neurology, vol. 7, no. 11, pp. 1032-1043.

[8]   Daly, J.J., Cheng, R., Rogers, J., Litinas, K., Hrovat, K. & Dohring, M. 2009, "Feasibility of a new application of noninvasive brain computer interface (BCI): a case study of training for recovery of volitional motor control after stroke", Journal of Neurologic Physical Therapy, vol. 33, no. 4, pp. 203.

[9]   Devanne, H., Lavoie, B.A. & Capaday, C. 1997, "Input-output properties and gain changes in the human corticospinal pathway", Experimental Brain Research, vol. 114, no. 2, pp. 329-338.

[10]   Do Nascimento, O.F. 2005, Movement-related cortical potentials, Center for Sensory-Motor Interaction (SMI), Department of Health Science and Technology, Aalborg University.

[11]   Dobkin, B.H. 2004, Neurobiology of rehabilitation.

[12]   Donchin, E., Spencer, K.M. & Wijesinghe, R. 2000, "The mental prosthesis: Assessing the speed of a P300-based brain- computer interface", IEEE Transactions on Rehabilitation Engineering, vol. 8, no. 2, pp. 174-179.

[13]   Endres, M., Heuschmann, P.U., Laufs, U. & Hakim, A.M. 2011, "Primary prevention of stroke: Blood pressure, lipids, and heart failure", European heart journal, vol. 32, no. 5, pp. 545-555.

[14]   Gerstner, W. & Kistler, W.M. 2002, Spiking Neuron Models: Single Neurons, Populations, Plasticity, 1st edn, Cambridge University Press.

[15]   Gillen, G. & Burkhardt, A. 2004, Stroke rehabilitation : a function-based approach, 2nd edn, St. Louis, Mo. : Mosby,.

[16]   Hebb, D.O. 1949, The Organization of Behavior: A Neuropsychological Theory, New edition edn, Wiley, New York.

[17]   Jackson, A., Mavoori, J. & Fetz, E.E. 2006, "Long-term motor cortex plasticity induced by an electronic neural implant", Nature, vol. 444, no. 7115, pp. 56-60.

[18]   Jackson, P.L., Lafleur, M.F., Malouin, F., Richards, C. & Doyon, J. 2001, "Potential role of mental practice using motor imagery in neurologic rehabilitation", Archives of Physical Medicine and Rehabilitation, vol. 82, no. 8, pp. 1133-1141.

[19]   Kennedy, P.R., Bakay, R.A.E., Moore, M.M., Adams, K. & Goldwaithe, J. 2000, "Direct control of a computer from the human central nervous system", IEEE Transactions on Rehabilitation Engineering, vol. 8, no. 2, pp. 198-202.

[20]   Kleim, J.A. & Jones, T.A. 2008, "Principles of experience-dependent neural plasticity: Implications for rehabilitation after brain damage", Journal of Speech, Language, and Hearing Research, vol. 51, no. 1, pp. S225-S239.

[21]   Krepki, R., Blankertz, B., Curio, G. & Mueller, K. 2007, "The Berlin Brain-Computer Interface (BBCI) --- towards a new communication channel for online control in gaming applications", Multimedia Tools Appl., vol. 33, no. 1, pp. 73-90.

[22] Langhorne, P., Coupar, F., Pollock, A. 2009 "Motor recovery after stroke: a systematic review." Lancet Neurology. vol. 8, no. 8, pp. 741-54.

[23] Mrachacz-Kersting, N., Fong, M., Murphy, B.A. & Sinkjær, T. 2007, "Changes in excitability of the cortical projections to the human tibialis anterior after paired associative stimulation", Journal of neurophysiology, vol. 97, no. 3, pp. 1951-1958.

[24] Mrachacz-Kersting N., Kristensen, S.R., Niazi, I.K. & Farina, D., 2012, "Precise temporal association between cortical potentials evoked by motor imagination and afference induces cortical plasticity", Journal of Physiology, Vol. 590, No. 7, pp. 1669-1682.

[25] Müller-Putz, G.R. & Pfurtscheller, G. 2008, "Control of an electrical prosthesis with an SSVEP-based BCI", IEEE Transactions on Biomedical Engineering, vol. 55, no. 1, pp. 361-364.

[26] Neuper, C., Scherer, R., Wriessnegger, S. & Pfurtscheller, G. 2009, "Motor imagery and action observation: Modulation of sensorimotor brain rhythms during mental control of a brain-computer interface", Clinical Neurophysiology, vol. 120, no. 2, pp. 239-247.

[27] Pavlides, C., Miyashita, E. & Asanuma, H. 1993, "Projection from the sensory to the motor cortex is important in learning motor skills in the monkey", Journal of neurophysiology, vol. 70, no. 2, pp. 733-741.

[28] Pfurtscheller, G. & Neuper, C. 1997, "Motor Imagery activates primary sensorimotor area in humans", .

[29] Rebsamen, B., Teo, C.L., Zeng, Q., Ang Jr., M.H., Burdet, E., Guan, C., Zhang, H. & Laugier, C. 2007, "Controlling a wheelchair indoors using thought", IEEE Intelligent Systems, vol. 22, no. 2, pp. 18-24.

[30] Roy, F.D., Norton, J.A. & Gorassini, M.A. 2007, "Role of sustained excitability of the leg motor cortex after transcranial magnetic stimulation in associative plasticity", Journal of neurophysiology, vol. 98, no. 2, pp. 657-667.

[31] Sejnowski, T.J. 1999, "The book of Hebb", Neuron, vol. 24, no. 4, pp. 773-776.

[32] Soekadar, S.S.R. 2011, "Brain–Computer Interfaces in the Rehabilitation of Stroke and Neurotrauma" in Systems neuroscience and rehabilitation Springer, Tokyo, pp. 3-18.

[33] Stefan, K., Kunesch, E., Benecke, R., Cohen, L.G. & Classen, J. 2002, "Mechanisms of enhancement of human motor cortex excitability induced by interventional paired associative stimulation", Journal of Physiology, vol. 543, no. 2, pp. 699-708.

[34] Stefan, K., Kunesch, E., Cohen, L.G., Benecke, R. & Classen, J. 2000, "Induction of plasticity in the human motor cortex by paired associative stimulation", Brain, vol. 123, no. 3, pp. 572-584.

[35] Truelsen, T., Piechowski-Jóźwiak, B., Bonita, R., Mathers, C., Bogousslavsky, J. & Boysen, G. 2006, "Stroke incidence and prevalence in Europe: a review of available data", European Journal of Neurology, vol. 13, no. 6, pp. 581-598.

[36] Vidal, J.J. 1973, "Toward direct brain-computer communication.", Annual Review of Biophysics and Bioengineering, vol. 2, pp. 157-180.

[37] WHO 2012, Cardio vascular diseases (CVD's), Fact sheets, WHO. http://www.who.int/mediacentre/factsheets/fs317/en/index.html.

[38] Wolpaw, J.R., Birbaumer, N., McFarland, D.J., Pfurtscheller, G. & Vaughan, T.M. 2002, "Brain-computer interfaces for communication and control", Clinical neurophysiology, vol. 113, no. 6, pp. 767-791.

[39] Ziemann, U., Paulus, W., Nitsche, M.A., Pascual-Leone, A., Byblow, W.D., Berardelli, A., Siebner, H.R., Classen, J., Cohen, L.G. & Rothwell, J.C. 2008, "Consensus: Motor cortex plasticity protocols", Brain Stimulation, vol. 1, no. 3, pp. 164-182.

[40] Ziemann, U. 2004, "TMS induced plasticity in human cortex", Reviews in the neurosciences, vol. 15, no. 4, pp. 253-266.

About the Author

Imran Khan Niazi was born in Mianwali, Pakistan, in 1981. He received the B.Sc. degree in Electrical engineering (specialization: Biomedical Engineering) from the Riphah International University, Islamabad, Pakistan, in 2005, and the Masters in Biomedical Engineering from University & FH Luebeck, Luebeck, Germany in 2009. In 2009, he joined the Center of Sensory Motor Interaction, Health Science Technology Department, University of Aalborg, Aalborg, Denmark as a PhD fellow under the supervision of Professor Dario Farina and Head of Department Associate Professor Kim Dremstrup. His academic research interests are rehabilitation, neurophysiology and signal processing. His PhD research topic was Brain computer interface for rehabilitation of stroke based on movement related cortical potentials.